Whole: A Pocket Guide to Finding Happiness in ALL Aspects of Your Life!

ISBN-10: 0692813720
ISBN-13: 978-0692813720

Printed in the United States of America

Whole

A Pocket Guide to Finding Happiness in ALL Aspects of Your Life!

Dr. Kate Nguyen, PharmD, IHC

Praise for Whole

Whole: A Pocket Guide to Finding Happiness in ALL Aspects of Your Life! encompasses exactly what I believe the author sets out to give you.

An introspective, inspirational exploration and comprehensive guide to being a healthier, happier person. *Whole: A Pocket Guide to Finding Happiness in ALL Aspects of Your Life!* by Kate Nguyen incorporates everything from mindfulness to financial planning to chronic conditions to eating local organic foods in a helpful and never preachy way. Kate Nguyen is real and thought provoking, she speaks from the heart, draws you in, takes you on her journey and gives you the steps to start, restart, or continue a journey of your own.

Nguyen lays out a straightforward strategy for attaining a more mindful, healthier life. Each chapter focuses on a different aspect of a holistic approach to happiness. The guide clearly states the author was once on a less mindful path herself, and it effectively uses her journey to a more enlightened state as an example throughout the text. This helps make the guide relatable and compassionate.

The chapters are well organized, making it easy to go back and refer to specific concepts, which make for a quick read. The language is simple and has a good rhythm without venturing into the trap of becoming either simplistic or esoteric. However, the book does a good job of making suggestions of how to slowly and systematically incorporate the ideas so change happens gradually and is sustainable.

A perfect guide for those who truly seek health and happiness, it is a practical guide which brought on a gamut of emotions for me—tears, smiles, laughter, ah ha moments, and I even caught myself doing the 478 deep breathing while reading it.

It is a thoughtful guide about taking responsibility for one's own life and particularly for one's own health and happiness. Nguyen offers the story of her own healing journey and discusses how she became empowered. Each honest story ends with the hope things can improve and it is really possible to change one's life for the better. The chapters are short and easy to digest. However, the simplicity and brevity make the book easy to rush through. It would be best to pause, think deeply, and truly accept each concept. There are numerous concrete examples to move quickly from theory to practice. The reader who diligently follows the path on their own journey will likely be taking a very wise step in the right direction.

Read. Appreciate. Apply.

~Rebecca King, RN, MSN, MPH, MBA, PhD

To Grandpa, for your structure, good health, and prosperity.
To Grandma, for your laid-back way of life.

Acknowledgements

Thank you to the following people for helping me make this book possible:

My dear friends, Guy and Ka, for being very enthusiastic first editors.

My brothers, Tom and Huu, and my friends, John, Jenny, Vicky and Julianne, and my colleagues, Maureen, Carmela, Alex, Kali and Jenni, for your words of encouragement and enthusiasm.

My friend, Tu, for the great photo.

Amanda Filippelli, for loving the book and for stellar editing and design work!

CONTENTS

My Grandparents..1

My Own Enlightenment...5

Preventing Chronic Disease..9

Plan. Progress. Enjoy..13

Nutrition...17

Exercise...21

Critical Numbers...23

Mindfulness...25

Relaxation..29

Sleep..31

Career..33

Financial Planning..35

Support System...39

Re-Evaliuate & Re-Balance Your Personal & Professional
Development..41

Thrive Wholly, Slowly, Safely & Surely..............................45

A Note From the Author

If you have any doubts that optimal health and happiness are worth investing in, the first few chapters of this book should melt those doubts away. Even better, you should be filled with inspiration, empowerment, and joy by the end of this book! If you read this book with an open mind and heart and take actions appropriately, it can transform your life in an amazing way!

My Grandparents

I was raised by my grandparents since I was one year old. They were my parents. When I was fourteen, my Aunt Loc and Uncle Don sponsored my grandparents, three brothers, and me so that we could come to the United States from Vietnam. I'm very grateful for my family, especially the relatives who welcomed, housed, and helped me get through the first few years of hardship in the U.S. My biological mother, her husband, and my other half brother and sister still currently reside in Vietnam.

After just a few years of living in the U.S, Grandma began falling off her bed in the early mornings, or off the sofa she was napping on during the day. These falls were followed by confusion and a headache. I later learned that these episodes were mini-strokes. Before long, Grandma had a major stroke, which debilitated her for the last fifteen years of her life.

My grandma also had osteoporosis, a disease in which the bones break easily, so every time she tried to walk again, to rehabilitate from the stroke, she would fall and break some bone, like her wrist. This made her too scared to try and walk again. As a result, she was either in a wheelchair or in bed for fifteen years, totally dependent on others to care for her, especially at the nursing home she resided in.

The stroke and osteoporosis stripped Grandma of her freedom (and her loved ones' of their freedom for a while too) to enjoy life to the fullest. This was very heartbreaking for her husband, me, and her other loved ones, like her eight children and many grandchildren.

What a domino effect! We would have loved to see her hang out with us, smile, laugh, and talk much more!

Grandpa, on the other hand, was pretty much independent until about two weeks before he passed away. He'd cook and pack delicious Vietnamese food, and take the bus to go see Grandma almost every day for those fifteen years. By the time Grandma passed, both of my grandparents were in their nineties and had been married for at least seventy-five years.

The main difference that I observed between their lifestyles was that Grandpa was much more active than Grandma, physically and mentally. They both ate pretty well; mostly fresh whole foods (vegetables, fruits, protein, and grains). Grandpa would walk or bike me around to church, school, parks, beaches, and our neighbors' houses. He also taught me how to swim in the ocean, which I still love to do! He didn't have any fancy gym equipment. He just stretched often and tried to maintain balance through naps and resting, prayers and mindfulness, through socializing, chores and work. He also loved reading and learning new things. This helped Grandpa maintain much of his mental sharpness up until the two weeks before he passed.

What I've learned from my grandparents' lives is that it is possible to live a long and healthy life, and that consistent healthful habits are key. As Aristotle said, "We are what we repeatedly do. Excellence is not an act, but a habit." Also, good health gives us the freedom to do things we enjoy, even simple things like walking!

My Own Enlightenment

I used to feel trapped and helpless, riddled with all kinds of ailments including idiopathic (no known cause) chronic urticaria (itching and hives all over my body), lower back pain, dry eyes, seasonal allergies, vitamin D deficiency, carpal tunnel syndrome, depression, UTIs, and lactose intolerance.

Although I was never diagnosed with depression by a physician (I used to try to hide this dark side of myself), I remember going to bed at night, many times thinking, "I hope I'll be dead in the morning so I don't have to deal with all the stress and suffering. Nobody really cares about me." Sure, there were quite a few significant stressors in my life, like helping three sets of parents and six siblings logistically, emotionally and financially, along with adapting to the American culture, learning a new language, putting myself through seven years of college including pharmacy school, and having a high-stress job. But, little did I know, chronic stress contributed greatly to my depression, which also had a lot to do with my perspective and level of mindfulness. I always had something external to blame for my depression, a victim mentality, and many times, I felt alone despite having quite a network around me.

So, how is it that I've been able to find health and happiness?

Practically all of my conditions have disappeared. I've been disease-free and medication-free for many years! I used to go to all kinds of healthcare practitioners in hopes of healing, especially for the urticaria and allergies. As a former practicing pharmacist and having experienced many complaints about medications and side effects, especially when taken long-term, I didn't want to take any chances. I was also concerned about the increased risk of autoimmune diseases (diseases in which the body attacks itself) due to these conditions. So, I slowly but surely made lifestyle changes to free myself from these chronic, idiopathic conditions so that I could thrive!

All of this has inspired me to write this book, to help inspire and empower others to own their health and happiness so they may live a free and prosperous life. The body has an amazing ability to adapt and heal when given even half a chance! Most importantly, balance is key for healing and staying well long-term.

Preventing Chronic Disease

For me, one of the biggest reasons to stay healthy is to avoid having to take medications. The side effects of medications, drug-drug interactions, and drug-food interactions can be limiting and frustrating. For example, drugs like levofloxacin and ciprofloxacin, the meds I used to take for my UTIs, can cause tendon rupture. Some antidepressants interact with foods like chocolate, red wine, and aged cheeses. A medicine for blood clots called warfarin interacts with dark leafy greens. Dairy adversely affects some antibiotics. Alcohol also interacts with many medications, and grapefruit can't be consumed while taking certain cholesterol and blood pressure medications.

So, yes, you could have much less freedom with food (and life!) when you're on meds. If you're a foodie like me, this is a huge deal! Plus, dark leafy greens are the most nutritious group of veggies so it becomes even harder to improve our health without them! They're practically my happy pills!

We must remember that although government agencies and pharmaceutical companies try their best to make prescription medications as safe as possible, there have been cases where approved medications have been withdrawn from the market due to unexpected harm or even deaths.

The bottom line: All medications and supplements have risks and benefits. Some medications definitely have their place, and if it weren't for the medications that controlled some of my symptoms, like itching hives all over my body, I wouldn't have been able to function. Medications bought me time to make lifestyle changes.

One should always weigh the pros and cons with their physicians and pharmacists so as to make informed decisions. Sometimes, when the benefits outweigh the risks, medications can help us buy time to make lifestyle changes to heal before getting off the medications with the help of our physicians. I've definitely seen this happen in my health coaching clients too!

Also, being sick is expensive! How did you feel the last time you had a short-term illness like a cold or an injured ankle? Do you remember how debilitating it can be when your body is missing a part or not functioning well? Imagine what it'd be like to have long-term or lifelong medical conditions...

Maybe you don't have to imagine. If you haven't had a costly illness yourself, talk with those who have. I have personally known people in their early thirties, forties, and fifties who have suffered from chronic medical conditions, like strokes and heart attacks. Some have even died of these conditions. Because of how heartbreaking this is, I've changed my career to health coaching to be more on the front line, helping to prevent this potential vicious cycle!

Having a chronic illness can cost a lot of money, time, and potential chronic stress, causing a domino effect since stress affects almost everything related to our health and wellbeing. Some common chronic medical conditions that you've probably heard of are heart disease, cancer, type II diabetes, arthritis, lower back pain, infertility, and depression. The good news is that most common chronic medical conditions can be prevented or even reversed! We really can enjoy a long and happy life! Just like almost anything else worth investing in, it takes some planning.

Whole

The ultimate reason to keep simple and stay healthy is so we have more time, money, and freedom to best serve each other and continue to do the things we enjoy for a long time to come. Benjamin Franklin once said, "An ounce of prevention is a pound of cure." The aim is to invest some resources, like time and money, on keeping well now, being proactive, so we won't have to spend much on curing or dealing with our own or even our children's illnesses in the future. I've found that being proactive can reduce stress tremendously and increase reliability.

So, by now, you're probably thinking, "Okay, okay, sold! What can I do to look good, feel good, and prevent most medical conditions for most of my life?"

Plan. Progress. Enjoy.

"It is good to have an end to journey toward, but it is the journey that matters in the end."

-Ernest Hemingway

I pick activities that I like, or I find ways to like what I do. This has helped me a lot to stick with things long-term! Plus, this is way better for my health and happiness. For example, to make cooking more fun, I play my favorite music and take short dancing breaks.

Now that I've captivated you, here's the juicy details on what I've been doing:

Write down or type up long-term SMART goals and positive motivators. SMART stands for Specific, Measurable, Attainable, Realistic, and Timebound. I place this sheet on my coffee table so I can see it every day until the changes I've made have been well integrated into my life and my goals have been achieved.

I write down or type up specific plans to reach these long-term goals and set aside specific blocks of time in my calendar to work on each regularly.

For example, one of my SMART goals is to reduce my body fat percentage to 21% by December, 2016. My motivators are to become more toned and stronger. My plan is to do weight training and martial arts on Mondays, Wednesdays, and Fridays for thirty minutes each, from 5:00pm to 5:30pm. I've scheduled these on my calendar.

I use the SMART goal method in many areas of my life, including the ones below.

Time Management – Balance Structure with Flexibility and Spontaneity

I have daily and weekly schedules with specific amounts of time allocated for routine essential things, like meals, exercise, and winding down, as well as a list of major projects, aspirations, and passions in order of priority. This way, I can just go down the list, achieving one or two items at a time. I also schedule non-routine things on my calendar, especially things that take longer than fifteen minutes to do. This has helped me tremendously with prioritizing and setting boundaries or saying no to things that are not important to me so I can stay focused on the things that are.

Look, there are always things to do and people to help or hang out with, so I ask myself three questions regularly: Can I afford the money and time it takes to do this? What are pros and cons? Am I spending most of my time and money on things and people that I value?

I also try to balance my time spent on a screen versus real-life experiences.

I schedule and take "health days" to recharge (so I almost never take sick days), and sometimes I just want to allow myself to be spontaneous on these days, doing more things that I enjoy, sometimes with my loved ones! A balance of structure and spontaneity is important to me, and keeps me healthy and happy.

De-Clutter, Clean & Organize – Make Your Home an Everyday Oasis

Clutter can drain energy and decrease efficiency. For example, I might not remember what I have and end up buying more of the same things and then can't find the things I need. I schedule to do a "brief de-clutter" and house cleaning every month on my calendar and a "thorough de-clutter and organization" every year, which involves donating clothes, shoes, and other household items that I've not used in the past couple of years. I organize things in categories, which helps me a great deal with efficiency and saves me money and time. Once I've designated a slot in my home for a category, it doesn't take long to start putting things there once I've purchased them. And the more organized and clean I keep things, the less daunting the scheduled cleaning and de-cluttering feels, and the more I can enjoy and relax every day!

Also, I don't wear street shoes in my house. Keeping my house clean helps tremendously with my allergies and minimizes my exposure to unwanted chemicals from the street and outside environment. I also keep my house well ventilated by airing it out regularly.

Nutrition

I've learned at least a hundred dietary theories (and I've forgotten most of them!), but this is the one that I follow: About 25% of my daily food consumption comes from fresh and whole fruits, vegetables, protein, and whole grains. I consume dark leafy greens almost daily, like kale, collard, chard, dandelion, spinach, bok choy, or mustard greens. The other color that I enjoy at least weekly is orange, like carrots, butternut squash, pumpkin, yams, and oranges. These help keep my immunity strong to fight off bacteria and viruses. Outside of these two staple groups of fruits and veggies, I strive for as many colors and as much variety as possible.

Some of my protein choices are plant proteins like beans, lentils, and soy. Some have good healthy fats in them, like fish and walnuts. I also consume natural sources of probiotics regularly, like yogurt and fermented vegetables. I try to buy organic or local as much as possible. Everything recycles so I try to support minimizing chemicals and treating animals (especially the ones I consume) and our earth with respect. I use olive oil for most of my food preparation, and I only eat out about twice a week.

I've never counted calories. I've focused heavily on quality and how nutritious and whole the foods I consume are instead. I also ensure that I spice my foods well, like with onion, garlic, pepper, turmeric, curry, ginger, cilantro, or Thai basil, to make them tasty without adding much sugar (if at all!) or salt. When we eat mostly whole foods (at least 80%) consistently, our bodies should become good at telling us when it's gotten enough of something or what it needs more of. I've never heard of anyone overeating dark leafy greens, have you?!

I also drink about thirteen cups (about 100 oz.) of water a day. I sip small amounts throughout the day, and since my body's been trained to get this amount of water, it often signals to me that I'm thirsty. I've learned about my community tap water via www.ewg.org/tap-water and use a filter that's certified to remove contaminants.

I rarely drink alcohol because I don't like the taste of most natural or whole brands, so the immediate pros don't outweigh the cons for me. Plus, alcohol has calories, which I'd rather get from tasty whole foods. I'll occasionally have sangria made with a pinot noir and fresh fruit, like oranges. And no, I do not need alcohol to enjoy social gatherings. I enjoy socializing just fine without any alcohol!

I make time for food planning at least once a week (yes, I schedule this on my calendar!). I have a menu of dishes that I like and associated ingredients to help me with efficiency. This has saved me a lot of time and money! Not to mention, it's helped keep me healthy, which helps me save even more time and money long-term, and most importantly to me, the freedom and ability to do things I like because I'm not debilitated by disease.

Exercise

My exercise routine includes many types of exercise: Cardio every day for at least thirty minutes, like brisk walking, swimming, dancing to my favorite music, martial arts, or running. Strength training (all major muscles) three times a week, like weight training, yoga, or Pilates. I also take brisk walks outside for at least twenty minutes on most days of the week, all year round, to get sunlight and fresh air. I used to have a vitamin D deficiency but have brought it back to normal since I started walking outside. I really enjoy my routine and it makes me feel good and strong! I warm up and cool down before and after every routine to prevent injuries and discomfort.

I also stretch every couple of hours and strive for proper posture regularly, especially when sitting a lot at my job. These breaks help prevent aches and pain from underuse or overuse of my muscles and joints. I also rest my eyes regularly by looking far (at objects twenty or more feet away), closing them, and blinking (the natural way our eyes moisturize themselves).

Among numerous other benefits including more energy, consistent and various exercises (cross-training) help us stay functional long-term so that we can continue to do necessary daily living things and hobbies with ease.

Critical Numbers

These are the numbers currently used by U.S. mainstream healthcare providers to predict risks for chronic diseases: BMI (Body Mass Index), LDL (bad cholesterol), HDL (good cholesterol), TG (fat), blood sugar, blood pressure, BMD (bone density), and vitamin D.

I stay within the normal range for these numbers. Also, I minimize fat around my waist. It's best to ask your primary care physician about what your numbers should be since they can vary depending on your specific medical record.

I check most of my numbers at least every two years to see exactly where I am so I know what I need to focus more on (if any) while not ignoring other areas. We don't want to fix one issue and end up with another! We need to focus on the whole person, not just parts and pieces. Everything interrelates so as we consistently eat healthier, exercise, manage stress in a healthier way, and acquire a balanced life, all of these numbers should normalize. For example, regular dark leafy greens consumption, cardio exercise, and minimizing highly processed carbohydrates and sweets should help improve most of these numbers tremendously.

Mindfulness

"The mind is a powerful tool. It can enslave us or empower us. It can plunge us into the depths of misery or take us to the heights of ecstasy. Learn to use the power wisely."

-David Cuschieri

We can use our minds to our advantage in so many ways. Have you heard of the placebo effect in drug studies? The placebo pills are the non-drug sugar pills in medication studies. A good percentage of people heal or improve their medical conditions when taking a placebo by just thinking that the placebo is the medicine that can help them! This is why studies are done to ensure that medicines actually work beyond this placebo-mind effect.

I practice mindfulness daily, both formally and informally. Defining mindfulness is not easy. In a nutshell, it's slowing down a little and being in the present, paying full attention, and making the most out of whatever I'm doing. The informal form could be anything I do throughout the day, like walking or washing my hands. The more mindful I've become, the more interesting and the more enjoyable my walks have become. I'm amazed at the variety in nature, like the cloud formations and colors in the sky, the trees, the birds and their singing, and even insects (as long as they don't crawl on me!). Also, the more mindful I am, the more grateful and uplifted I feel. Gratitude definitely contributes to my good health and bliss!

The formal form, meditation, comes when I actually sit down or lay down in a quiet place and zone inward to cultivate great stuff, like peace, compassion, kindness, humility, and love. It helps ground me and realigns me with my most important values, and connects me with the comforting higher being(s) beyond us that many call God. Also, meditation has helped me to be kinder to myself and more grateful for my body. This has also helped me cultivate even more authenticity (toward myself and others), which contributes greatly to optimal health and joy as well!

Before sharing negative things with others, I think about whether doing this will benefit me or the listener(s) first. If not, and I decide not to do anything about it or have no control over it, then I try not to share, and I surrender to the Universe.

Mindfulness has also helped change my perspective on most things, from looking at the glass as half empty to half full, seeing the positives in almost everything! Amazing! For example, I've begun viewing stressors as opportunities rather than threats. I've basically acquired a lot of optimism! Marcel Proust once said, "The real voyage of discovery consists not in seeking new landscapes, but in having new eyes." Okay, how about both new landscapes and new eyes? Yes, please!

Whole

"Seek and you will find."

Relaxation

I use free, easy, and convenient ways to relax. For example, I use deep breathing multiple times a day. It helps me calm down instantly. I also take mind vacations through guided imagery several times a day using my mind or computer screen saver image to take me to my happy place, like through awesome mountains or to the ocean.

Most of us can't afford but about a few weeks of leisure travel per year, so it's really important that we take timeouts and enjoy every day for long-term health and happiness. Plus, why not?!

sleep

My favorite thing to do! I strive for eight hours of good quality and restorative sleep nightly. One thing that helps me to sleep is unwinding for at least half an hour by watching a sitcom or something relaxing before bedtime. Yes, regular laughter is essential! Another way to relax is by using the 478 Deep Breathing Technique to help me fall asleep faster when needed. I just inhale while counting for four seconds, then hold for seven seconds, then exhale while counting for eight seconds. A very long breath!

Some other things that help me to have good restorative sleep are a sound machine or quiet environment, a comfortable temperature and darkness in the bedroom, consistent exercise, healthy nutrition (of course!), like avoiding caffeine (in coffee, tea, chocolate), especially a few hours before bedtime, consuming dark leafy greens regularly, and minimizing processed carbohydrates and sweets. Other things that I do throughout the day help my sleep as well, like being outside in daylight for at least twenty minutes a day and practicing mindfulness and relaxation at least a few times a day.

Career

I've traded more than half of my annual salary for joy. I wholly believe we can really live long, prosperous, and free lives, so I've allowed myself to be more on the front lines to help others through health coaching. I've followed one of my biggest passions! I'm very grateful for my pharmaceutical knowledge as this has uniquely helped me and my clients as well.

If you hate your job, especially if it's a high-stress one, this might be detrimental to your health, especially in the long run. Stressful jobs can leave us with serious, debilitating medical conditions later in life that no amount of money can save us from! For long-term optimal health and happiness, it's important to pick a career that you like, or to find ways to like what you do and stay balanced.

I was very scared at first, resigning from a stable pharmacist position to give myself time and energy to soul-search. I also had to spend a lot of time and money on additional education in Integrative Health Coaching and made practically no money at first as a health coach. But slowly, I've built a career that I love. Although I have a list of passions, I've picked the most practical and realistic one and have pursued it first. I had to do a lot of planning, including financially to ensure comfortable living despite making less money. But all my hard work has been very worthwhile!

Financial Planning

I have a budget. I know roughly the total of both my monthly incomes and my expenses. Having my finances in order has given me the freedom to follow my passions and maintain a comfortable and enjoyable lifestyle. I balance living now and saving for comfy living later in retirement.

Experience and knowledge from multiple resources tells me it's wise to have a cushion of at least one year's worth of expenses and to save at least 10% of your annual salary for retirement in the forms of 401K, HSA (Health Savings Account), ROTH, and a traditional IRA. But most importantly, I stick closely to my budget and only spend less than what I earn or have at all times.

Although I've managed my money well for the most part, I have made a couple of unwise financial decisions, and these have cost me a lot of time and money! To bounce back, I've lived by these two principles: I don't spend the money I don't have (especially debts with high interest rates, like credit cards) and I stop trying to make money quickly. I've acquired more patience when it comes to saving and investing! I'd rather diversify, take less risk and earn less more steadily over a longer period of time than to take a whole lot of risk and potentially lose a big chunk over a short term. Again, I balance risks and benefits here. Setting SMART goals financially has also helped me dig myself out.

There are quite a few budget worksheet templates online that you can use to create your own, including on bank websites. There are also financial advisors who can help with things like picking mutual

mutual funds for your 401K, HSA, IRAs, etc. I have a financial advisor! My first one was from a bank that I had my first checking account with and I met my current advisor at a community finance class years ago.

Whole

Here are some things you should consider including on a budget worksheet template that you can use Excel to create:

Account 1 Income
Account 2 Income
Savings Total

Pending Big Purchases
Max House Purchase
House Down Payment

Retirement Accounts & Balances

Add up your total monthly expenses. Then subtract them from your monthly income. The leftover is what spending cash you have!

Monthly Expenses
Mortgage/Rent
AC/Furnace Filters
Humidifier Filters
Water Filter
Utilities (Internet,
Electric, Gas, Water)
Food/Eating Out
Haircut
Gas/Carwash
Car Insurance
Gifts
Health Insurance
Cell Phone
Coffee
Loan Payments
Tolls
Vacation/Hobbies/Gym
Miscellaneous

Support System

Although I have many relatives and know many people, there are only a select few that I totally trust, confide in, and keep in touch and laugh with on a regular basis. These precious, long-term friendships are mutual and we're very grateful for each other. We've been there for one another through the peaks and troughs of our lives. We've comforted as well as celebrated each other.

For optimal health and happiness, it's very important that we have at least a couple of people whom we trust, confide in, cheer us on, fuel us, and give us constructive feedback so we can continue to thrive and stay healthy and happy. We, humans, are finite in time, money, health, and other resources. So, it's really important that we set boundaries with ourselves and others, including our loved ones, to minimize unnecessary stress and to make time for self-care. This helps us continue to serve for a long time to come. Regular chronic stress caused by toxic people that is not dealt with in a healthy way can increase our risk for debilitating and costly chronic medical conditions, which can cause us to become a burden on our loved ones or society. So, in essence, taking care of ourselves regularly is taking care of others, especially in the long-run. No one knows our limits as much as we do our own. So, communicating and enforcing these limits and listening to our bodies are key to balance and long-term health and happiness.

Albert Schweitzer said, "At times, our own light goes out and is rekindled by a spark from another person." This is why it's so important to have genuine, positive, and supportive people in our close circles.

Re-Evaluate and Re-Balance Your Personal & Professional Development

I've found that I sometimes drift away from my important values or my callings, like when I swim in the ocean and the current pushes me where I don't intend to go. So, when I ocean-swim, I periodically check my landmarks to ensure I don't unintentionally swim too far away.

For example, I used to Facebook for at least an hour every day; time I could have used to write this book! This is why I re-evaluate when I feel imbalanced or when important things on my list or schedule are not getting done in a timely manner. Sure, this takes some time, but I'd rather take time to re-gain control of my life rather than feel out of control. We're happier when we are in charge of our own life.

Like Muhammad Ali said, "A man who views the world the same at fifty as he did at twenty has wasted thirty years of his life." I also enjoy growing and progressing, both personally and professionally. I ensure that I allocate enough time for both consistently! Some call this work-life balance and growth.

Some examples of personal development for me are things like improving my WHOLE health, style, finances, and hobbies further. I enjoy short reads on these subjects and implementing changes along the way. One example of improving my health further is to use more whole and natural external products, like skin moisturizers and cleansers. This is not only better for my health, but also for Mother Earth.

Professional development, for me, includes pharmaceutical and health coaching knowledge and skills. For example, I regularly read medical articles and inspiring articles on optimal health, happiness, and vitality to keep myself up-to-date with relevant information, honing my skills accordingly. SMART goals help me tremendously with making these changes happen. A moderate amount of growth and change keeps our senses and whole-person active, sharp, and happy!

Change and development ties back to the importance of the balance between structure and flexibility. If we want to stay healthy and happy, another way to see this is as a balance of being proactive in accomplishing our goals in this finite life while also "going with the flow." This balance helps us to both achieve our callings or passions while also enjoying the amazing surprises that life brings as well as a peace within!

Thrive Wholly, Slowly, Safely and Surely

It's important to note that the changes I've implemented into my healthful way of life I've made slowly and safely over a long period of time. It's been so worth the investment of my time, money, and effort! Now, I'm not only healthy physically, but also emotionally, mentally, and spiritually. But I'm still a work in progress and probably always will be!

I've replaced, "Why I can't," with, "How can I?" and this helps me honor my most important values, like my health and self-care. I'm amazed by the fun and creative solutions I've come up with! The secret to change, for me, is to focus much more energy on building the new than fighting the old.

When you decide to start making some changes to optimize your health and happiness, you might find that you need an accountability partner, a catalyst, someone to hold your hand through this process, at least for the first part of this awesome journey. There are health coaches out there that can be this person for you. You can check with your employer to see if health coaching is something they offer in your benefits package. Some employers now carry this benefit. If not, you can ask them to or find your own!

Happy owning YOUR WHOLE health and bliss. Believe and make it happen!

"Start by doing what's necessary; then do what's possible; and suddenly you are doing the impossible."

-St. Francis of Assisi

About the Author

Kate Nguyen acquired her Doctor of Pharmacy degree at Virginia Commonwealth University and practiced pharmacy for several years, where she evaluated, dispensed, and monitored many medication regimens as well as promoted healthful lifestyle behaviors to the community through patient education. After seeing so much suffering due to preventable chronic diseases (personally & professionally) and the associated healthcare costs, she started her quest for a wholesome and proactive approach to healthcare and discovered Integrative Health Coaching! Kate received her Health Coach training from Duke University and the Institute for Integrative Nutrition. As a certified Integrative Health Coach who has healed her own medical conditions by using a whole body-mind-spirit approach, Kate hopes to help people prevent and/or reduce the negative impact of many debilitating and costly chronic diseases on themselves as well as their caregivers. She has been partnering with people to work on healthy and long-term weight loss, stress management, mindful awareness, nutrition, physical activities, and other lifestyle changes for several years. Kate passionately wants to empower others to own their health and happiness so that they can save time, money, and have the most joy and vitality possible.

In addition to the routine activities mentioned in this book, she also likes to sing, dance, and might attempt to compose music one day! She also loves water and water sports and occasionally jet skis, kayaks, and stand-up paddleboards with her loved ones.

www.ingramcontent.com/pod-product-compliance
Lightning Source LLC
Chambersburg PA
CBHW070942280326
41934CB00009B/1986